WEIGHT LOSS FORMULA

WEIGHT LOSS FORMULA

CD&SP+RE+PR+QS&R= WL

Lose weight and belly fat within 30 days while loving the process

AVERY VANNS

WEIGHT LOSS FORMULA

LOSE WEIGHT AND BELLY FAT WITHIN 30 DAYS WHILE LOVING THE PROCESS

E-mail: projectselfdevelopment@yahoo.com

ISBN: 9781099786358

IMPRINT: Independently published

DISCLAIMER

No part of this publication may be reproduced or transmitted in any form or by any means, mechanical or electronic, including photocopying or recording or by any information storage and retrieval system, or transmitted by email without permission in writing from the publisher.

While all attempts have been made to verify the information provided in this publication, neither the author nor the publisher assumes any responsibility for errors, omissions, or contrary interpretations of the subject matter herein.

Weight loss formula proposes a fitness program and recommendations for the readers to follow. However, you should consult a qualified medical professional before starting this or any other fitness programs. As with any exercising or dieting programs, if you experience any severe discomfort you should stop immediately and consult your physician.

The views expressed are of those of the author alone, and should not be taken as expert instruction or command. The reader is responsible for his or her own actions.

Neither the author nor the publisher assumes any responsibility or liability whatsoever on the behalf of the purchaser or reader of these materials.

Any perceived slight of any individual or organization is purely unintentional.

TABLE OF CONTENTS

WEIGHT LOSS FORMULA..................................1

TABLE OF CONTENTS 6

INTRODUCTION 7

CHAPTER 1: DECIDING TO LOSE WEIGHT...13

CHAPTER 2: IMPORTANCE OF DIET AND MEAL PORTIONS...18

CHAPTER 3: THE POWER OF EXERCISING ..24

CHAPTER 4: PLEASURE REWARDS 35

CHAPTER 5: QUALITY SLEEP AND REST 42

CHAPTER 6: ACTION ITEMS.............................49

BONUS CHAPTER...53

CONCLUSION..56

INTRODUCTION

Jack sits alone in the dark on his couch comfortably watching a new season of Game of Thrones on his 40in LED flat screen television. He slowly scoops up a spoonful of ice cream into his mouth, as tears slowly trickle down his jaw to lose themselves in the hairy jungle of his beard. He then slowly swallows the soft, cold, and creamy spoonful of mouth-watering ice-cream which melts away steadily on his tongue. What is it that has made jack so sad? What has caused a 300lb man to be in such a pitiful condition?

Earlier in the evening when he pulled up in his driveway he saw something very worry-some; there was a pair of male and female running shoes on his 'welcome mat'. "It must be her brother's," Jack said to himself, as he casually opens the front door into his house. A stomach-twisting feeling gripped his body when he saw there were two glasses of wine half emptied on the countertop, and the horror movie 'lights out' playing on his TV. He said to himself, "her brother doesn't drink wine or watches scary movies, and who could she have over at 6:30 p.m. without calling to tell me." These were all the thoughts that flooded Jack's mind as he anxiously took off his shoes and slowly hung his coat.

"NO!" Jack heard his wife scream from the bottom of her lungs. Jack's already racing heart then felt as if it skipped two beats, and beads of perspiration began to form on his petrified body along with an army of goosebumps. He quickly stormed up the stairs towards the direction of his bedroom where the scream originated, only to see the door locked in the distance of his foggy eyesight. Without stopping he furiously rammed his shoulder on the door sending it flying open.

Fuelled with adrenaline and an instinct to protect, Jack barged through the door to see his wife lying on the bed covered in sweat, whip cream, and chocolate syrup. Sarah, his wife, was seen handcuffed to their king size bed with her eyes rolled over in the back of her head and a bright and satisfactory smile on her face. "Sarah!" Jack shouted as the car keys fell out of his hand, and then in the corner of his eyes, he saw a man dressed in a robber's mask naked holding a bottle of olive oil. Both the masked man and Sarah were startled and could not move or utter a sound out of their mouth; they were caught red-handed.

Jack fell to his knees and enraged in anger; he shouted, "What's going on?" looking her squarely in the eyes. After many attempts to speak with a voice suppressed in deep emotions, she said, "This is my gym partner Thomas, he was the millionaire entrepreneur I was telling you about." Jack retorted, "Why? Why did you do this? Haven't I given you everything?" Then Sarah replied, "I've been telling you for years to go to the gym with me and take care of your body, but you wouldn't listen to me, and you got so fat to the point where I honestly stopped feeling any form of attraction for you. I'm sorry but if you had just listened this wouldn't have happened." After hearing her reply, Jack shouted, "Both of you get the hell out of my house."

Thomas, without hesitation, quickly pulled the handcuff around Sarah's hand, and they both hurriedly put on their clothes and ran out of Jack's house without looking back. Jack meanwhile enraged with mixed emotions on his knees could do nothing more than punch his fist into the ground, yelling and screaming in anger to release his pent up emotions.

Fast forward to jack sitting on his couch sadly eating his almost finished bowl of ice-cream. He thought about losing weight and getting his body back into beast mode. Then a deep desire to lose weight and prove to his cheating wife he is capable of taking control of his life stroke him like a bolt of lightning. Infused with a deep desire and definiteness of purpose, a new light gleamed in Jack's eyes. He then stood up, the tears stopped, and he threw the bowl of ice-cream in his garbage bin, then grabbed his old dusty running gears, stepped through the front door and took action.

Although this scenario is fictitious, I sincerely hope that no one and anyone who is reading this has to go through that level of pain to make a change in their lives. Maybe you're like me, I was facing obesity and going to the gym, only to stop after two weeks because I wasn't getting the results I wanted fast enough. For many people losing weight seems impossible and for others, they don't want to go through the pain of exercising, push their bodies to the limit, or miss eating their favourite foods. I understand I was that guy, the thought of exercising and dieting can only be described as a fish trying to climb a tree. However, for me, the harsh truth came when I realized that it was that way of thinking that got me to the point of being overweight and unhappy with my body.

I knew there had to be a way to lose weight without going through extreme workouts and excruciating diets. I spent months researching, reading books, experimenting with different workout routines to find the answer, or a set formula I could use to lose weight at a moderate pace and enjoy the process simultaneously. My determination led me to discover a single formula that helped me to lose over twenty pounds in three months. With that knowledge, I decided to write a very short and concise book which could help anyone to solve their weight loss problems.

I'm not a nutritionist, scientist, fitness coach, or a self-development guru. I'm just a regular everyday guy who wants to help as many people as I possibly can to lose weight and get their dream body, and I know you want that too.

This book was written short and concise so there isn't any difficulty in finishing the book and implementing what you have learned. If you are a procrastinator who will only read a few pages of the book, and you will not implement what you have learned then this book cannot help you. If you expect to go half in, do the bare minimum and get the results you're looking for this book won't help you. This book is for action takers and committed warriors who will implement what they have learned to get the body they deserve, and I want that person to be you. So let's dive in and get you losing weight now!

CHAPTER 1: DECIDING TO LOSE WEIGHT

You bought this book so you can turn your life around, congratulations on making the right decision. So many people want a change in their lives but prefer to sit down with their wishful thinking, complain and do nothing about their situation. I applaud you for being the one percent of action takers who refuse to settle, unlike the ninety-nine percent of whiners and complainers who are silently drowning in the sea of mediocrity.

You deserve the body of your dreams, you know you have what it takes to put in the hard work and get the things you want in life, otherwise, you wouldn't have bought this book let alone be reading it. What I want you to recognize is that your life will only change, when you make the decision that you want to change to make your life better. If you only read the book and you don't implement the knowledge you've learned, you're no better off than someone who didn't spend their hard working money to invest in themselves. Please read this book multiple times and take action; it is the only way you'll get the solutions to your problem.

"The most important investment you can make is in yourself."

___ Warren Buffett

The hardest part of losing weight or doing anything worthwhile in life is when you have to make the tough decisions that will make you feel uncomfortable, and sticking to those decisions even when the journey is hard, painful, challenging, or disappointing. It is only when you make a decision that your life begins to change. Making a commitment to yourself will ultimately allow you to become successful in anything you set your mind to, and this is why it is the most crucial part of losing weight.

"Commitment is what transforms a promise into reality."

___ Abraham Lincoln

I was once a procrastinator who always took the easy route and made excuses about why I couldn't exercise. My bad habits led me to stop taking care of my body, and I ate unhealthy foods which caused my weight gain. Later I realized that the decisions I made had more negative consequences where I developed stretch marks and a severe stomach ulcer, which could have been prevented if I ate healthy foods and exercised regularly. However, you have invested in this book, and it shows yourself and me that you have the right mentality for living a better quality of life.

THE POWER OF A DECISION

People usually decide out of inspiration or desperation, where they are inspired by something or someone which motivates them to make a change, or out of misery where they are desperate to get out of their current situation. If you are in a desperate situation like I was then you know how painful it feels to look in front of the mirror and look at your body. It was out of desperation that I got the motivation I needed to exercise and diet, and by sticking to that commitment, I lost over twenty pounds in only three months. If I could do it, then you can do the same in your life.

The first thing you need to do is decide on how much weight you want to lose in a specific period of time. You can do this by writing it down in a book or journal and read it every day. Then you need to know your reason for wanting to lose weight, with that clarity you can endure all the pain and sacrifices that you'll have to make. I would like you to write down your why in the same book or journal, and read it daily to continually remind yourself why you are putting yourself through the pain and discomfort. Having clarity will be your anchor and purpose to continue on the path of weight loss.

My reason, for wanting to lose weight was so I could feel more confident with my body and to attract the opposite sex. Your reason might be different, but once you know you're why, you can endure almost any how. However, this is just the first step in transforming your body; the next step in the chapter that follows is taking care of your diet and eating healthy.

"Your why, when coupled with determination is like a light in the dark cave of uncertainty and self-doubt, it will enable you to take action and find your way."

___ Avery Vanns

CHAPTER 2: IMPORTANCE OF DIET AND MEAL PORTIONS

Having a healthy diet is by far one of the most essential parts of weight loss if not the most important, and it is something that many people take for granted. In my country there is an old saying, "You are what you eat," and this couldn't have been said any better. The type of foods and the quantity you consume is what ultimately decides your overall health and body weight.

Weight gain is very simple and easy to understand. The more unhealthy foods rich in fats, sugars, and oils you consume and the less physical activity you engage in, the more likely you are to gain weight. The opposite for weight loss is also true; if someone eats a well-balanced diet including meals from the five food groups, exercises regularly and consumes those foods in small portions it is less likely that person will become overweight. This knowledge is common sense, there is no need to pay money to listen to any health professional to give you that basic information.

A general rule of thumb to know the appropriate food portion for you is to cup both of your hands together, and the amount of food that can fit within your palms will show you how much food you should be consuming. To implement a smaller meal portion, you should start by reducing the size of your meals gradually every day until you reach a comfortable limit. When I just started what I did was eat out of a smaller dish and gradually reduced my food portion as a way to sort of trick my brain into thinking that I'm eating the same amount of food, because the smaller portion would also fill up the dish.

Next, you should drink lots of water to where your stomach feels full after you finish your meals so that you can compensate for a large amount of food you would normally consume. For example, if you eat a small sandwich of bread, boiled eggs, sliced tomatoes and lettuce, then you should drink one or more glasses of water to fill up your stomach. This hack works by filling up your stomach with water which will eradicate any feeling of hunger you might be feeling. It works wonders in reducing your temptations to eat more food and makes the process of reducing your food intake a lot easier and bearable.

All of this might sound a little too simple, but the truth is often simple. If you stop and think about it, eating less and consuming healthy foods not only help in weight loss, but it also makes your body feel and look better, increases your mood, and boosts your productivity. Choosing to live a healthier lifestyle should become your top priority and not a hard decision to make. Eliminating junk foods, sodas and artificially flavoured beverages, and processed food should be something to explore or at least reduce consuming them in your diet.

SIMPLE DIET HACKS

- Remove junk food out of your home
- Buy groceries and cook your meals based on the five food groups
- Refrain from eating most of your meals at restaurants
- Make a diet plan on the weekends (preferably on Sunday), with the meals you will prepare and eat

at specific times (breakfast, lunch, and dinner) for each day of the week

- Reduce sugary artificially flavoured beverages, sweet pastries and salty foods in your diet
- Drink mostly water throughout the day and real fruit juice made with real fruits and/or vegetables
- Get an accountability partner(s) and share your diet goals to ensure you stick to your diet
- Read books or go online and research on diets that can help with weight loss
- Implement an 80/20 rule. 80% consists of a clean and healthy diet consisting of the foods from the five food groups, and 20% are your favourite not so healthy and junk foods in small portions
- Avoid eating then sleeping
- Eat your meals in a small dish at home. If you have to eat at a fancy or fast food restaurant order the small size meal.

Reducing the portion size of your meals is very important and should not be taken for granted. Without you eating healthier and consuming less food, it will take you a significantly longer time to lose weight, and if you see no results chances are you will stop, become discouraged and eventually go back to your old eating habits. I want you to discipline yourself to stick to a clean diet from the five food groups and delay immediate gratification of eating junk foods. Adapting this good habit into your life is what will ultimately decide whether or not you'll live a healthy lifestyle and build a strong foundation for weight loss.

I sincerely hope you'll take this chapter seriously and take charge of your health. You only get one vehicle to carry you through life, and that's your body. I suggest you take care of it like it was the only car you would ever get in your entire life, surely you would put the best oils possible and give it the best servicing and maintenance money can buy. So why not do the same for your body and make your health a top priority? Why not put the best foods money can buy and give your body the best treatment possible? My friend, you and you alone, are responsible for your health so please take care of it.

The following chapter is the stepping stone of good health and is the backbone of weight loss, which is none other than exercising.

CHAPTER 3: **THE POWER OF EXERCISING**

For most people pushing their bodies to the limit and facing all the stress and pain that comes with exercising isn't something they look forward to. However, many people cannot see that nothing in life comes easy and you have to work hard for what you want. Exercising is no different; to achieve the body of your dreams in becoming healthy, exercising is a crucial ingredient in achieving this goal.

It is possible for some individuals to do nothing and have a well-shaped body based on their genetics, but even for those people if they don't take care of their health, even genetics won't be able to keep their physique.

I want you to drill into your head the importance of physical activity; if you are overweight or obese, you will not lose weight by just sitting on a couch and imagining yourself with a flat stomach or six pack abs. It would be best if you conditioned your mind to get into the habit of exercising and put in the hard work, which is the best way to get the results for the body you want.

I did not like exercising one bit, the constant muscle aches during and after exercising were undoubtedly my, "I can't take this anymore" moment. I was sick and tired of not being able to run for 30 seconds without my lungs feeling like they were about to burst. So, I started to run for 30 minutes, 3 times a week until I could go an entire hour of jogging and love every second of it.

The first thing I did was to decide on a time convenient for me to wake up and start exercising. Exercising schedules will be different for each individual based on their lifestyle and circumstance. A person working a 9-5 job could wake up at 5 a.m. and exercise for 30 minutes to an hour, while a college student may have to exercise in the evenings around 5 p.m. based on how their classes and study timetable are scheduled. It's vital that you set a time, which is convenient for you each day.

Unfortunately, on some days you will not be able to exercise, and that's ok; as you can reschedule your workout for another day during the week. Initially when you're just starting to exercise it's essential that you stick to the time you choose 100% until exercising becomes your routine. The objective is to make exercising a habit, so you no longer have to think about doing it or force yourself to make the tough decision to exercise or procrastinate.

Most people think that exercising will never get easier because of all the pain they are feeling. However, I promise you it will, especially when your body has adapted to the tiny muscle tears. Eventually, the excruciating pain will stop. It is crucial that you add some variety to your exercising regiment because if your body gets used to you exercising a particular way all the time, you will stop losing weight.

It would be best if you also challenged yourself to come up with a variety of exercises and workout routines to prevent your body from adapting fully, which will cause you to stop losing weight. Here are some of the things that you can do to add variety in your workout:

- Increasing the duration of the workout
- Increasing the intensity and pacing of the workout
- Implement new exercising routines
- Implement a fun sporting activity with a friend

The second thing I did was to choose a suitable location where I could exercise with no distractions, which would prevent me from doing my workout routines. For example, I did my workout inside my room or at the gym when the weather was bad. What I advise you to do is to choose a spot in your house that is spacious enough, and do indoor exercises at your convenience. Exercising indoors eliminates any excuse you might have to exercise if there is bad weather outside.

For outdoor workouts, it's wise to choose a location that's near your home and in an area that is safe and hazards free. Outdoor exercising can be done in ideal places such as the park, your neighbourhood, or your backyard. After choosing a suitable location, next, consider the type of workout, which is ideally suited for your weight loss.

MAKE EXERCISING FUN AND EXCITING

Exercising can be very fun depending on the workout routine you engage in and who is doing the workout with you. Personally, for many people including myself who can't afford to maintain a gym membership, get a workout buddy, or hire a personal coach, it can be extremely difficult to find the willpower and self-discipline to get in the mood to exercise. Hence, I found one main exercise that was fun and rewarding, which I could easily do without thinking, having a workout partner or personal coach, and that exercise was jogging.

Jogging is one of the most rewarding exercises because you get a full body workout and burn many calories without having to spend a dime. What more could you ask for? So what I did was to jog 2-3 times a week until I worked my way up to four, and then I incorporated my other workout routines with jogging, such as shadow boxing, squats, push-ups, sit-ups, football, etc.

Also, it is important that you choose fun sporting activities you love and incorporate them into your workout routine. So on the days when your willpower is low, and you don't possess the motivation to exercise, you can easily engage in that fun sporting activity as a means of exercising. Some of the fun sporting activities you can choose from include; swimming, dancing, tennis, table tennis, basketball, netball, baseball, cricket, football, rugby, etc. Choose a specific day in the week for your sporting activity and have fun, as a bonus it will make you look forward to exercising even more.

A simple hack that will help you to stick to your workout and follow through is to get an accountability buddy. This person can be anyone that will hold you accountable for exercising which could be a friend, family member, or your intimate partner. What this does is to have someone in your life that will support your exercising commitment, to ensure that you complete your workout each week especially on the days you want to sleep in or skip a day and procrastinate.

EXERCISING RITUALS

Now, it's time to take action, but before that, there are some things you need to have to get the best out of your workout. Some of these include:

- A light running shoes for your daily jogging and workout
- A bottle of water to prevent dehydration
- A sweater/ hoodie and sweatpants for cold weather conditions
- A phone or watch to keep track of time
- A towel or rag to dry yourself

To begin your exercising routine, all you need to do is start exercising and forming the habit. Start by scheduling the days and time you are comfortable with, then prepare ahead of time. Preparations may include buying a new pair of running shoes, buying exercising gears or machines, choosing a workout partner, or hiring a fitness coach, sign up for a gym membership, etc.

Next, if you choose to do your workout in the evenings or at night make sure you have completed most of your work based related and/or family based activities first, then you should exercise. This habit is important because if you have work or other things to do regarding your family, and you prioritize exercising this can cause you to neglect those other aspects of your life which can have a lot of negative consequences. So exercise when you are free from urgent or important tasks.

If you decide to exercise early in the morning, set the alarm either using an alarm clock or mobile device and place it away from your bedside or in a next room where you can still hear it. This method works by forcing you to get up out of your bed to stop the alarm, and it also removes any temptations to hit the snooze button for, "just five more minutes." After waking up if you feel thirsty ensure that you drink a little water, be careful not to drink a lot which can cause you to develop stitches, which are very uncomfortable when jogging.

Next, you should get a bottle of room temperature water, put on your workout gears, and head to the gym, or a spot either in your house, at your workout area, or somewhere outside. Then begin doing some warm-up exercises to stretch your muscles and warm up the body before engaging in any vigorous exercise. Warming up will prevent any injury or harm to your body from exercising, such as serious muscle aches and torn muscles or ligament, etc.

Warm-up exercises can be found on YouTube. For example, fitness blender.com and Howcast are great sources for warm-up exercises and other health and fitness content. Also, fitness apps such as Freeletics is also great for having a steady workout routine and hiring a fitness coach; I recommend this to anyone who is on a budget so they can hire a cheap fitness coach to guide them through their weight loss process. Ensure that you get your own set of warm-up exercises, which you'll do each day before your workout begins.

Finally, after you have completed your warm-up, you should immediately start exercising. If you're someone who is just starting, ensure that you begin slowly at a pace you are comfortable with at first. Do not push yourself too hard or overstrain, as this could potentially cause serious harm to your body. Go at your own pace, whether you are doing your workout solo, or in a pair or group, remember you have nothing to prove by tearing a muscle.

In the first two weeks of exercising, only exercise for 15-30 minutes three times a week. Remember, the aim is to form the habit of exercising, so there isn't any inner resistance, and you don't have to force yourself to exercise. It should become automatic to the point where you don't think about doing it, and it becomes effortless.

What helped me to better understand habit formation was a course on YouTube by Improvement pill called, "The Tamed course." Ensure you watch it before you exercise multiple times and stick to the information in the course. You will become better at habit formation for not only exercising but in almost any area of your life and also to overcome any addiction you may have.

After the two weeks have passed, you must increase the intensity and gradually the duration of your daily workout routine. Your new objective should then be to increases the duration until you have reached the hour mark and gradually increase the intensity of the workout also.

Always add variety to your workout, and find new ways to push yourself and stretch your comfort zone.

Note that the purpose of jogging is to burn fat and lose weight; it will not aid in bulking up. Other exercises like lifting weights, serves the purpose of bulking, so if you lose enough weight and your new objective is to gain muscle you will have to change your workout routine to match your goal.

Now we have covered exercising; the next step will aid you in forming the habit for the long term. In this next chapter is a powerful tool called Pleasure rewards.

CHAPTER 4: **PLEASURE REWARDS**

Everyone loves to get a reward after completing a very hard and challenging task, for pushing themselves to tap into their reserve energy and accomplishing great feats. It is for that feeling of, "I deserve this" that makes receiving a reward meaningful. Receiving rewards is a very pleasurable experience, and we as humans crave pleasure and run away from pain, which is the reason why a person would rather sit down and play video games all day than to workout at the gym.

Many people struggle with sacrificing instant gratification, where they give in to the immediate dopamine rush instead of making conscious long term decisions for their betterment. This causes people to develop poor habits that consequently have more negative effects on their lives in the long term. Choices such as eating tasty junk foods and drinking alcohol, are just a few pleasures that make you feel good at the moment but has a lot of negative long term side effects, such as obesity and alcohol addiction which both destroys your health and family relationships.

In self-development or improving any aspect of your life, it will take a tremendous amount of work, commitment, discipline and courage to yield life-changing results. Depending on the change you are trying to accomplish it can be a very stressful and painful experience in sticking to that commitment and changing existing beliefs and bad habits. For example, take this scenario, a man or woman goes on a thirty-day challenge to wake up and exercise six times a week hoping to lose twenty pounds, and starts strong and vigorous in their workout for the first week, however, somewhere in the second week they will become discouraged and stop. Why do you think that happened? I'm sure you know someone who has done the exact same thing and ended up with the same result. I want you to think about it and develop your conclusion after you have completely read this chapter.

This chapter is the icing on the cake to help you solidify and engrain the habit of exercising, to where you look forward to completing your workouts. The concept is straightforward; it is rewarding yourself with a pleasurable reward at the end of each workout session. It works by encouraging your brain to want to exercise, where it associates completing a session of a workout as being pleasurable. What I want you to do is after you finish exercising, reward yourself with a small treat you enjoy on the days when you exercise. Rewarding yourself should be done until you feel as if you look forward to exercising, then you will no longer need the reward at that point.

TAKE DELIGHT IN WORKING HARD AND PLAYING HARD

The rewards you should give yourself need to be something you love. For example, it could be having a small bowl of ice cream, having a warm bath soaked in red wine or milk, playing video games, receiving a full body massage from your partner and for adults having sex with your significant other. These are just a few of the many pleasures you can give to yourself after exercising. Nothing, however, is more powerful, pleasurable and rewarding than having sex.

Sex is the most pleasurable experience, and reward you could ever give to yourself because it not only feels good; it also relieves stress, burns calories, and aids in developing a stronger bond with your partner as a bonus. I do not under any circumstance condone sexual activities between children or underaged teenagers; it is only for adults and adults only. However, in relationships convincing your partner to have sex with you can be a little challenging, so an open discussion and negotiation is the best place to start.

This method of reward will work best if you and your partner both agree to have sex on the days when you exercise and directly after the exercise has been completed. The pleasure from sex will drastically improve your drive to exercise, where you will look forward to that feeling of immense pleasure and sexual gratification whenever you will be doing your workout. It can also be very exciting to have sweaty animalistic sex and sex in the shower; I'll leave you and your significant other with that to think about as a means of spicing things up.

Rewarding your partner after having sex can reinforce and encourage more sex in your lives, so it's a win-win situation for both of you. Having convenient sex might not be possible for most single persons, so I recommend that you find something else that you enjoy doing or having. For example, if you love eating sweet treats like a bowl of ice cream, or having a doughnut; ensure that you do it sparingly and in moderation. Be mindful that eating too much will set you back on your hard work.

REWARD YOUR WAY TO GOOD HABITS

Habit reinforcement is the foundation of changing your life, and it is something that will take both time and energy for the change to happen. Without giving yourself a reward that will encourage change then it will take you a lot more time, effort and trials before getting the results you want, so please take this seriously.

What I recommend you do is write down a list of rewards you enjoy, and have a variety of pleasurable rewards, so you don't become tired of having or doing the same things. For example, on the three days of exercising you can have a small bowl of ice cream on the first day, receive a full body massage on the second day, and have sex on the third day after your workout and switch it up the following week. I guarantee you will reach a point where you're coming out of bed excited to exercise.

It is also important to know that it's ok to slip up and make mistakes, not all the time will you be able to give yourself a reward based on your circumstance or the type of day you're having. However, what's important is that you try to get a reward the other time you're exercising so you don't fall off track and blame yourself for not owning up to your commitment. This applies to diet, exercising and sleeping; it's ok to mess up a few times. Once you get back to doing the right things as soon as possible, then you won't have to worry about procrastinating or breaking your commitments to yourself and others.

Pleasurable rewards are the key to forming the habit of exercising and anything else in your life you want to change. Change isn't something that can be easily forced, but change is easily encouraged when it is paired with pleasure.

Now that we have covered how to form the habit of exercising, next, to the secret to losing weight that many people overlook, and that is quality sleep and rest.

CHAPTER 5: QUALITY SLEEP AND REST

At this point, you should have acquired the knowledge you need for dieting, exercising and pleasurable rewards, there is one last component of the equation for simple weight loss, and that is quality sleep and rest. Sleeping and resting your body is a very crucial part of weight loss because your body requires time to make the necessary repairs to burn fat effectively and develop your muscles.

Without resting your body, you may as well did not exercise because you will be doing more harm to your body than good. Getting quality sleep of about seven hours or more each day is highly beneficial to your overall health, as it not only recharges and repairs your body; it also improves your health and builds your immune system etc. Too many people take their sleep for granted, and they destroy their health and well-being. I implore you to make getting quality sleep a top priority in your life not only for weight loss but also for your overall health.

Imagine how tired you would feel after a long and hard day's work, and going home all you want to do is kick off your shoes, take a shower, eat, watch a movie and lie in your bed as soon as possible. Now imagine after that hard day's work, all you could get is four hours' worth of sleep and then your day starts all over again. Every day it's the same amount of sleep and the same amount of work or sometimes more; how long would it take to burn out or end up in the hospital worst case scenario? Do not permit yourself to sacrifice your sleep for work or other pleasures, ensure that you get a good nights' rest every day.

When exercising, if you don't get enough rest not only will you slow down your progress of attaining the results you want, you risk developing severe injuries. To prevent this from ever happening you should try to get at least 6 hours, an average of 7-8 hours, and a maximum of 9-12 hours' worth of quality sleep each night as a rule of thumb.

By this time you have heard me mention quality sleep often and you might wonder what it means to get quality sleep. Quality sleep is simply uninterrupted sleep in a pitch black room free from light and awful noises. Ensure that your room is without lights and noises when you retire to bed at night, as these can potentially ruin the quality of sleep you receive. A simple hack to block out unwanted sounds and lights is to wear a sleep mask and earmuff when you go to bed at nights.

Placing a bottle or glass of room temperature water at your bedside is very important if you get thirsty during the night. This recommendation is so that you won't have to ruin your sleep when you feel thirsty, by having to go to the kitchen frequently to have a drink of water. Be careful not to drink too much water, as this will cause you to have to wake up and go to the bathroom frequently. Frequent urination can also potentially ruin the quality of your sleep. If you do happen to wake up thirsty during the night, drink a small quantity of water that is enough to quench your thirst.

EXERCISING AND RESTING YOUR BODY

As I stated in this chapter, it is crucial that your body gets the rest it needs to repair itself after exercising to prevent injury. Getting adequate rest should be implemented throughout your lifetime of exercising, and especially when you are just starting. Please take this seriously, because I know from personal experience of sprain ankle and groin injury, the toll it can take on your body and the damages that can happen if you do not rest your body after exercising.

What I recommend is when you are just starting, exercise up to three times a week and rest for the other four days without doing any workout. As you exercise for more than a month, you can go up to four or five days a week and rest for two days without doing any exercises. You might worry that this strategy will not give you any results, and you need to exercise as much as possible to lose weight, which is completely wrong. Your body is like a machine, and even machine needs rest, or it will eventually crash and burn, unable to work efficiently.

Once you have done everything in the previous chapters, then you have nothing to worry about or fear. Here is my routine that I used initially in the beginning stages; I went to bed 9 o'clock every night, then I woke up at 4 o' clock in the morning and exercised until 4:45 a.m., three days a week. For the remaining four days I rested my body, and I slept for seven hours every day, which made me feel energized and well rested.

SLEEPING TO GET THE BODY OF YOUR DREAMS

Many people do not sleep at the same time each day, and I was guilty of also doing this many times. However, you must condition yourself to sleep at the same time each day to regulate your circadian rhythm, which is known as your sleep/wake cycle. It is simply when your body has a specific time when you want to sleep and a specific time when you wake up in the morning. When you regulate your circadian rhythm by going to bed the same time each day, it will make falling asleep easier to where you'll want to sleep the same time, and you'll be able to wake up without an alarm.

Ensure you go to bed at the exact same time every day and wake up at the same time, you should have a routine that gives you 7-8 hours of sleep. If you are someone that sleeps in the day time all the information in this chapter applies to you as well, you just need to adjust it to suit you when you're sleeping in the day time. On the days you don't exercise, you need to ensure that you are sleeping the same 7-8 hours, or if you can even more.

There is one thing you must never do before sleeping, and that is to eat right before you go to bed. When you're asleep your body isn't able to fully break down and digest the food in your stomach, so your body will store the majority of the food as fat. It slows down your digestion progress which enables you to gain more weight from storing the food as fat, and it can potentially lead to heartburn. Promise yourself you won't do this under any circumstance; it's better to go to bed hungry than risk gaining weight. Always eat 3-4 hours before bedtime which gives your body enough time to digest and break down the food consumed fully.

Sleeping is very important so don't take it for granted, coupled with a clean diet and constant exercising you will start losing weight. The formula for weight loss is simple, and it goes:

Clean Diet and Small Portions + Regular Exercising + Pleasurable Rewards + Quality Sleep and Rest= Weight Loss

Weight loss formula= CD&SP + RE + PR + QS&R= WL

And with that formula, hard work and commitment you will lose weight and get the body you know you deserve.

CHAPTER 6: **ACTION ITEMS**

CHAPTER 1: DECIDING TO LOSE WEIGHT

Action item:

1. Write down in a book or journal why you have decided to lose weight, and what is the positive impact it will have on your life

2. Write down the amount of weight you want to lose in x amount of month. Ensure it is achievable or your brain will come up with all the reasons not to exercise. Example, (I want to lose 10 pounds in 2 months)

3. Read aloud every day once before you go to bed and once when you wake up, so it's all you can think about when you first wake up

CHAPTER 2: IMPORTANCE OF DIET AND MEAL PORTIONS

Action Item:

1. Gradually reduce eating junk foods
2. Reduce the portion size of all your meals in half at the beginning and later on into quarters. E.g., Use a smaller dish or plate to eat your food and buy smaller size meals at the restaurant
3. Decrease your sugar intake, for example, stop drinking sodas. Instead, drink lots of water with every meal, lightly sweetened tea and drink real fruit juice as an alternative to drinking sodas or artificial flavour juices

CHAPTER 3: EXERCISING

Action Item:

1. Using the calendar app on your mobile device or a blank calendar set the date and time when you will be exercising each week at your convenience
2. Choose the location where you will do your workout. E.g., your home, the gym, in your neighbourhood, at the park, etc.
3. Choose a partner(s) or fitness coach(optional) to help with your workout and also choose the

specific warm-up exercises and workouts that suit you and serves your weight loss goals

4. Prepare the day each day before by getting the necessary gears you'll need to exercise and place them at a location that is easy to find. E.g., buy new running shoes, sweat pants and a sweatshirt (optional), hoodie, a case of bottled water, etc.

5. Go to bed at a specific time each day to get 7-8 hours of sleep and set the alarm preferable in a different room where you can hear it, or away from your bedside so you can wake up fully without hitting the snooze button

6. Dress in your gears carry a bottle of water, phone/watch and head to the spot where you'll exercise. Ensure you do warm-up exercises first, then after you're ready to start exercising (for 20-30 minutes at the beginning stages)

CHAPTER 4: PLEASURE REWARDS

Action item:

1. Write down 3-6 pleasurable rewards you enjoy and can do readily in your notebook
2. Each day after your workout give yourself one of the pleasurable rewards from your list
3. After exercising has become a habit and you no longer have to think about doing it, then you can reduce your rewards and focus on forming another habit implementing the same principle

CHAPTER 5: QUALITY SLEEP AND REST

Action Item:

1. Ensure that you get an average of 7-8 hours of sleep each day
2. Go to bed at the exact same time each day
3. Choose set days during the week where you will not exercise and rest
4. Never eat and then go to your bed. Eat each day 3-4 hours before your bedtime so your food can be completely digested

BONUS CHAPTER

We've journeyed a long way together, and now that I've planted the weight loss formula in your head I know you'll take action and use it to change your life. However, I love to over deliver and I couldn't end this book without delivering huge value, so this chapter is me giving you additional help with your weight loss and life.

"Type the addresses below in YouTube to find the contents."

WARM-UP

- Fitness Blender: Easy Warm Up Cardio Workout
- Fitness Blender: Quick Warm Up Cardio Workout

RUNNING

- Howcast: How To Pick the Right Running Shoes
- Howcast: How To Get Started Running
- Howcast: How To Have Proper Running Form

- Howcast: How To Run In Cold Weather
- Howcast: 3 Common Mistakes

DIETING

- Howcast: How To Exercise Portion Control
- Howcast: How To Develop Healthy Eating Habits

SLEEPING

- BRIGHT SIDE: 8 Tricks to Sleep Better According to Athletes

PLEASURE REWARDS

- Improvement Pill: How Often Can You Slack Off? Q&A Episode #3

HABIT FORMATION

- Improvement Pill: How To Change Your Bad Habits- The Easiest Way

- Improvement Pill: Tamed Course

All the information you need is in this chapter, so I implore you to commit to never-ending growth and constant evolution to live the best possible life. I know how hard it is to take action and change your life. I also know that it's difficult to work, but nothing that comes easy is worth it, so remember that the next time you plan on sitting on the couch depressed, overweight and living a life of mediocrity scrolling on social media hoping that you'll get the motivation to make your life better.

Start right now do not wait on the perfect time or for the stars to align, work with what you have at your disposal and get your heart pumping and your soul alive again for true happiness comes from refusing to settle and challenging yourself to be better than you were yesterday.

"Change will come ONLY when the pain of staying the same is greater than the pain of change."

___ Dora Lee Scott

CONCLUSION

Congrats champ, you made it to the end, many people would have stopped reading, but you are not like them. Instead, you're an action taking badass who refuses to settle, and I'm proud of you. You've taken the initiative to change your life, and I commend you for doing so, not only will this book help you get the body you've longed for and dreamt about, by taking action this book is the tool for your freedom and immeasurable life transformation.

Don't wait, do not procrastinate and let this be just another book lost in your phone or computer, make a promise and commitment to yourself that you will follow this book's teaching and implement it in your life. I don't expect you to let this knowledge go to waste and just be useless information, I know you will put it to practice and lose weight, you know that too. I want you to make a commitment to yourself that you will take action and change your life. Add your name to the blank space below and read it aloud twice daily, once when you wake up in the mornings and when you retire to bed at nights.

"I _____ will commit to losing weight starting now to change my life and become the best version of myself. I will prove to any and everyone who has doubted me in the past that I am capable of taking control of my life and of my destiny".

Again thank you for purchasing this book and changing your life. Share this book with your family and friends or anyone you know who wants to lose the extra pounds and have the body they've always wanted. Now go and change your life and remember the sacrifice will be worth it.

If you have enjoyed reading this book and you feel excited, empowered, and you love the investment you made in yourself, then please go and leave a neutral, honest review for this book on Amazon and share your reading experience with the world☺. Also, continue shopping on the world's best retail store, you already know its Amazon.

If you have any questions, criticism or breakthroughs you would like to express, feel free to contact me directly at: projectselfdevelopment@yahoo.com.

www.ingramcontent.com/pod-product-compliance
Lightning Source LLC
Chambersburg PA
CBHW072119280526
45788CB00006B/2552